THE GRATITUDE JOURNEY

Discover, Embrace & Flourish

By La'Joi Carter

Introduction:

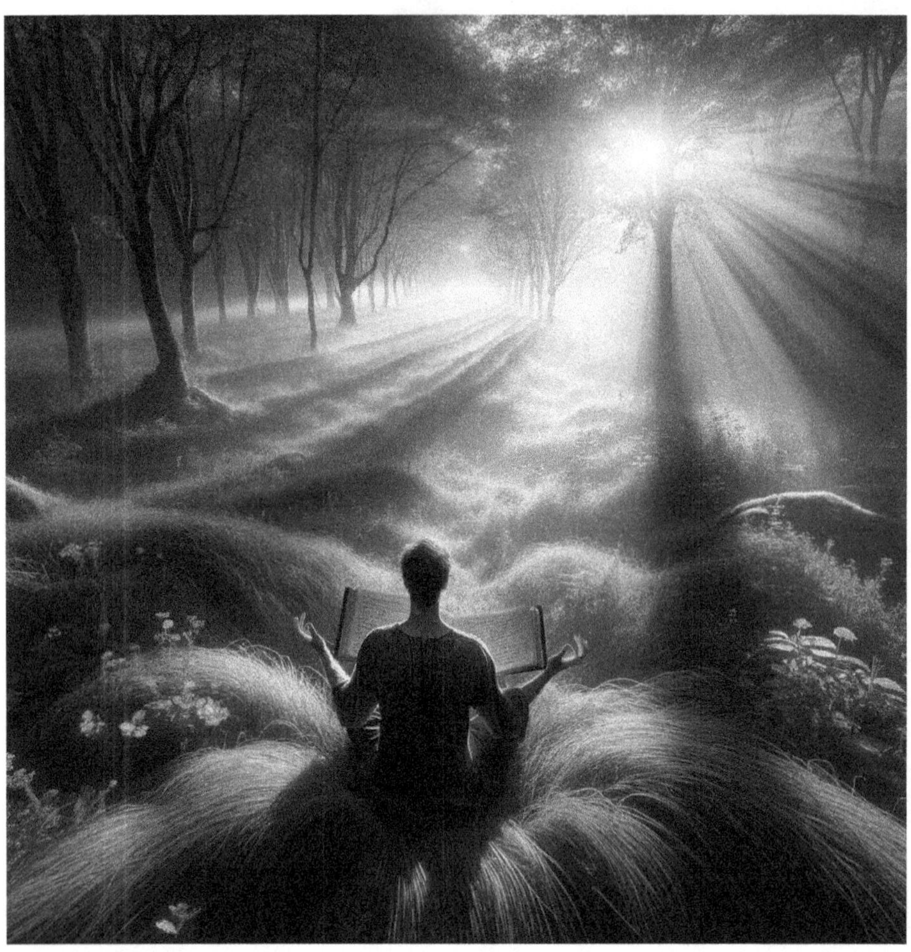

In a world filled with constant noise, distractions, and challenges, it's easy to lose sight of the simple yet profound treasures that enrich our lives every day. Amidst the hustle and bustle of modern life, there exists a timeless remedy—a powerful antidote to the chaos—that has the potential to transform our outlook, our relationships, and our very existence. This antidote is gratitude.

Welcome to "The Gratitude Journey: Discover, Embrace, and Flourish." Within the pages of this book, we embark on an expedition into the heart of gratitude—a journey that will illuminate the path to profound joy, fulfillment, and personal growth.

Gratitude is more than just a fleeting feeling of thankfulness; it is a fundamental orientation toward life—a lens through which we perceive the world and engage with our experiences. It is a deeply rooted appreciation for the abundance that surrounds us, from the smallest moments of beauty to the grandest blessings.

In this exploration, we will delve into the essence of gratitude, unraveling its mysteries and uncovering its transformative power. We will discover how gratitude is not merely a response to favorable circumstances but a deliberate practice—a way of being—that can be cultivated and nurtured, regardless of our circumstances.

Throughout these pages, we will explore the science behind gratitude, delving into the psychological and physiological benefits that it bestows upon us. We will examine practical techniques and exercises for cultivating gratitude in our daily lives, from mindfulness practices to gratitude journaling and beyond.

But our journey doesn't stop there. We will also explore how gratitude can be applied in the face of adversity, serving as a beacon of hope and resilience during life's most challenging moments. We will uncover its profound impact on personal growth, emotional intelligence, and relationships, as well as its ability to foster a culture of appreciation and generosity in our communities and workplaces.

Above all, "The Gratitude Journey" is an invitation—a call to embark on a transformative quest toward a life of deeper meaning, connection, and fulfillment. As we embark on this journey together, may you open your heart to the abundant blessings that surround you, and may gratitude become the guiding light that illuminates your path toward a life of joy, purpose, and flourishing.

CHAPTER 1: THE ESSENCE OF GRATITUDE

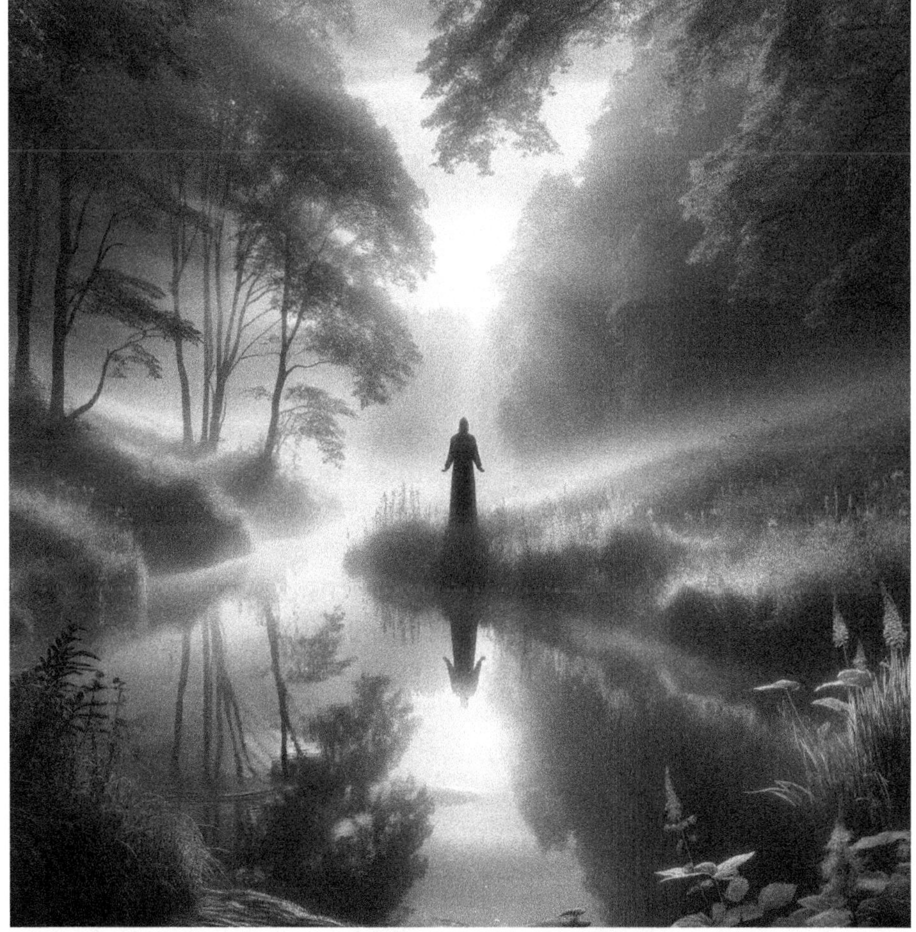

In the quiet moments of reflection, when the noise of the world fades into the background, we often find ourselves drawn to the simple but profound question: what does it mean to be truly grateful?

At its core, gratitude is a profound acknowledgment of the blessings, big and small, that enrich our lives. It is an attitude —a way of seeing the world through the lens of appreciation and abundance. Gratitude is not merely about saying "thank you" for the good things that come our way; it is a deeply rooted recognition of the inherent value and beauty in every moment, every experience, and every interaction.

But gratitude is more than just a fleeting emotion or polite gesture; it is a fundamental orientation toward life—a perspective that shapes how we engage with the world and interpret our experiences. It is the recognition that even in the midst of challenges and hardships, there is always something to be grateful for—a silver lining, a lesson learned, a moment of grace.

The essence of gratitude lies in its ability to shift our focus from what is lacking to what is present, from scarcity to abundance. It is a practice of reframing our perspective, choosing to see the glass as half full rather than half empty. In doing so, gratitude has the power to transform even the most mundane moments into opportunities for joy and appreciation.

But gratitude is not just a feel-good sentiment; it is also backed by science. Research in the fields of psychology and neuroscience has shown that cultivating gratitude can have profound effects on our well-being, both mentally and physically. Studies have found that practicing gratitude can increase feelings of happiness and contentment, reduce symptoms of depression and anxiety, and even improve physical health outcomes such as immune function and cardiovascular health.

So how do we cultivate gratitude in our daily lives? It begins with a shift in perspective—a willingness to pause, to notice, and to appreciate the beauty and abundance that surrounds us. It involves cultivating a sense of mindfulness, learning to be present in the moment and to savor the richness of our experiences. It means taking the time to reflect on the blessings in our lives, big and small, and to express heartfelt gratitude for them.

In the chapters that follow, we will explore practical techniques and exercises for cultivating gratitude in our daily lives. We will delve into the science behind gratitude, examining its profound effects on our mental, emotional, and physical well-being. And we will uncover the many ways in which gratitude can enrich our lives, from fostering deeper connections with others to enhancing our sense of purpose and meaning.

But perhaps most importantly, we will embark on a journey of self-discovery—a journey toward a deeper understanding of ourselves and the world around us. For in the practice of gratitude, we not only find joy and fulfillment but also a profound sense of interconnectedness—a recognition that we are all part of a larger tapestry of life, woven together by the threads of gratitude and love.

CHAPTER 2: CULTIVATING GRATITUDE

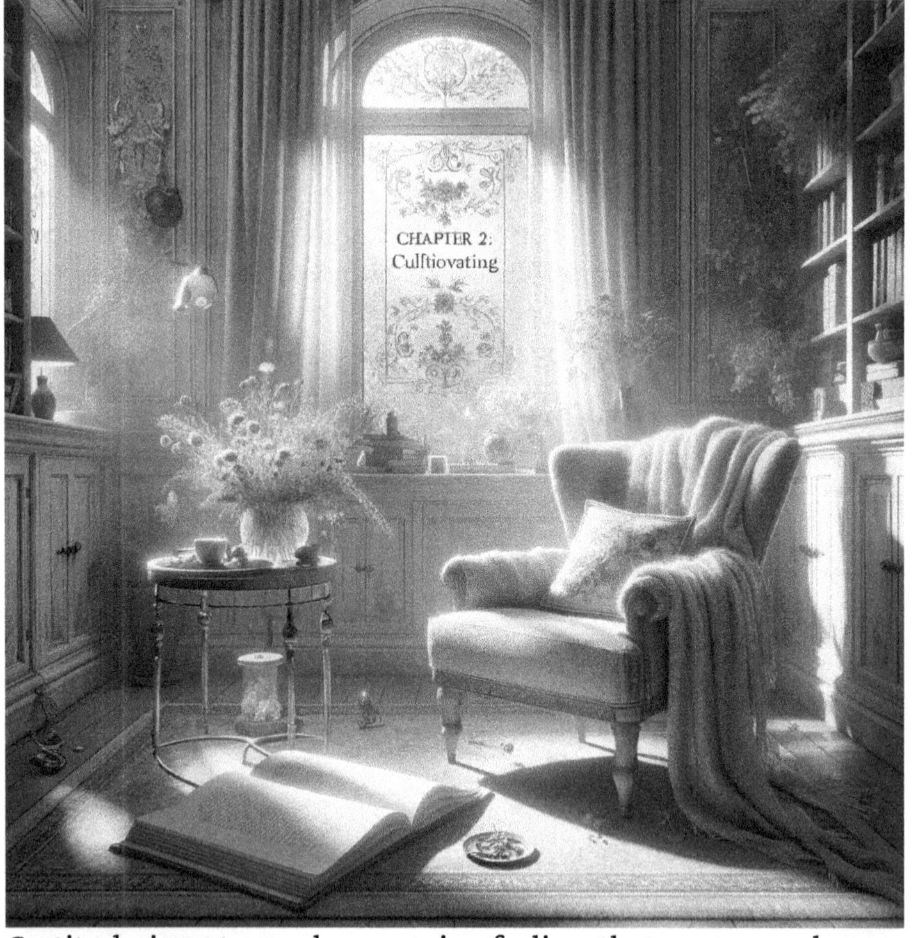

Gratitude is not merely a passive feeling that comes and goes;

it is a practice—an intentional choice that we make each day to acknowledge and appreciate the blessings in our lives. Cultivating gratitude is like tending to a garden; it requires patience, nurturing, and consistent effort. In this chapter, we will explore practical techniques and exercises for cultivating gratitude in our daily lives.

1. Mindfulness and Gratitude:

Mindfulness is the practice of being fully present in the moment, without judgment or attachment. By cultivating mindfulness, we can develop a deeper awareness of the abundance that surrounds us and cultivate gratitude for it. Try incorporating mindfulness practices such as meditation, deep breathing, or simply taking a few moments each day to pause and notice the beauty and richness of your surroundings.

2. Gratitude Journaling:

One of the most powerful ways to cultivate gratitude is through journaling. Keep a gratitude journal where you can write down three things you are grateful for each day. These can be simple pleasures, like a warm cup of tea or a beautiful sunset, or more significant blessings, like the love of family and friends. Writing down what you are grateful for helps to anchor your awareness in the present moment and reinforces a mindset of abundance.

3. Gratitude Rituals and Practices:

Create rituals and practices that help you to cultivate gratitude on a daily basis. This could be as simple as saying grace before meals, taking a moment to express gratitude before bedtime, or starting each day with a gratitude meditation or prayer. Find practices that resonate with you and incorporate them into your daily routine.

4. The Role of Gratitude in Relationships:

Gratitude is not only a solo practice; it also plays a crucial role in fostering deeper connections with others. Make it a habit to express gratitude to the people in your life—whether it's a heartfelt thank you, a handwritten note, or a small act of kindness. Cultivating gratitude in your relationships not only strengthens your bonds with others but also enhances your own sense of well-being.

5. Gratitude in Adversity:

While it may be easy to feel grateful when things are going well, true gratitude shines brightest in the face of adversity. When life throws challenges your way, take a moment to reflect on what you can still be grateful for—whether it's the support of loved ones, the lessons learned, or the resilience that arises from difficult times. Cultivating gratitude in adversity can help to shift your perspective and empower you to find meaning and growth in even the toughest of circumstances.

As you embark on your journey of cultivating gratitude, remember that it is a practice—a lifelong commitment to nurturing an attitude of appreciation and abundance. By incorporating mindfulness, journaling, rituals, and practices into your daily life, you can cultivate a deep sense of gratitude that enriches every aspect of your existence.

CHAPTER 3: APPLYING GRATITUDE IN CHALLENGE

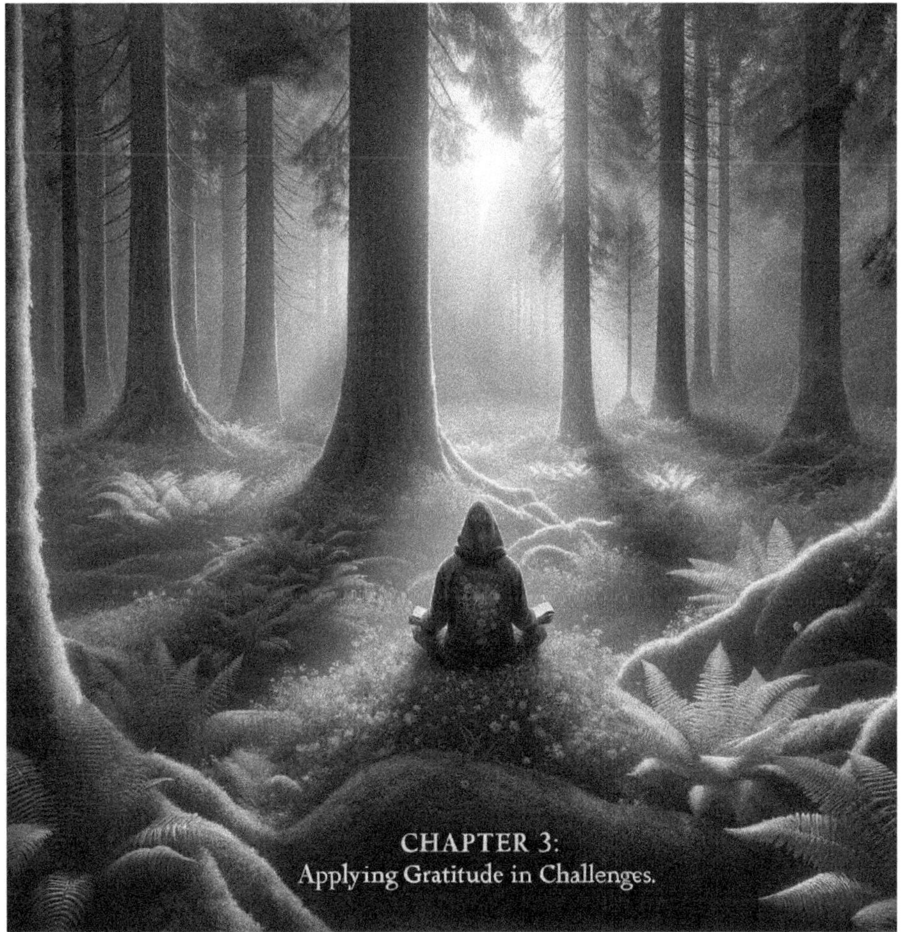

Life is a journey filled with ups and downs, twists and turns, triumphs and trials. In the midst of life's challenges, cultivating gratitude can serve as a guiding light—a beacon of hope and resilience that helps us navigate even the darkest of times. In this chapter, we will explore how to apply gratitude in the face of adversity and use it as a powerful tool for personal growth and well-being.

1. Finding Silver Linings:

Even in the midst of difficult times, there are often silver linings—lessons learned, unexpected blessings, moments of grace. Cultivating gratitude involves training our minds to look for these silver linings, even when they may be difficult to see. When faced with challenges, take a moment to reflect on what you can still be grateful for, no matter how small or seemingly insignificant.

2. Overcoming Negativity Bias:

As human beings, we are wired to pay more attention to negative experiences than positive ones—a phenomenon known as negativity bias. Cultivating gratitude involves consciously overcoming this bias and training our minds to focus on the positive aspects of our lives. Practice gratitude exercises such as gratitude journaling or gratitude meditation to counteract negativity bias and cultivate a more balanced perspective.

3. Gratitude and Resilience:

Resilience is the ability to bounce back from adversity and thrive in the face of challenges. Cultivating gratitude can enhance our resilience by helping us to find meaning, purpose, and strength in difficult times. When faced with setbacks, use gratitude as a tool to reframe your perspective, focusing on what you can learn and how you can grow from the experience.

4. Gratitude as a Coping Mechanism:

Studies have shown that practicing gratitude can have powerful effects on mental health, helping to reduce symptoms of depression, anxiety, and stress. When facing difficult emotions or situations, use gratitude as a coping mechanism to help regulate your emotions and find a sense of calm and peace. Focus on the things that you are grateful for, no matter how small, and allow gratitude to uplift and soothe your spirit.

By applying gratitude in challenges, we not only find strength and resilience but also deepen our appreciation for the richness and complexity of life. As you navigate the ups and downs of your journey, may gratitude be your constant companion—a source of light and inspiration that guides you through even the darkest of times.

CHAPTER 4: GRATITUDE AND PERSONAL GROWTH

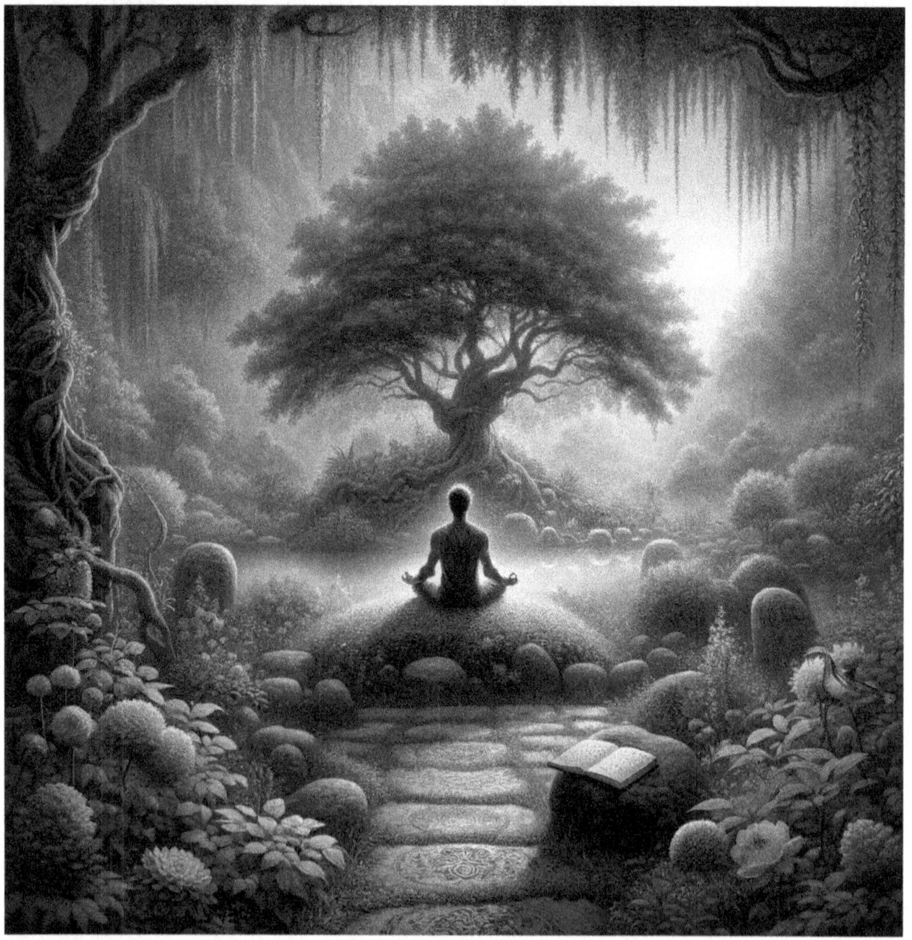

In the journey of life, personal growth is a constant

process of evolution—a journey of self-discovery, learning, and transformation. At the heart of this journey lies gratitude, a powerful catalyst for growth and development. In this chapter, we will explore how gratitude can fuel our personal growth and lead us to greater levels of fulfillment and well-being.

1. Gratitude and Self-Reflection:

Self-reflection is the cornerstone of personal growth, providing us with valuable insights into our thoughts, feelings, and behaviors. Cultivating gratitude can deepen our self-awareness and self-understanding, helping us to identify our strengths, weaknesses, and areas for growth. Use gratitude as a tool for self-reflection, reflecting on the blessings in your life and the lessons they hold for you.

2. Gratitude and Goal Setting:

Setting goals is an essential part of personal growth, providing us with direction and motivation to pursue our dreams and aspirations. Cultivating gratitude can enhance our goal-setting process by helping us to focus on what truly matters and what we are already blessed with. When setting goals, take time to reflect on the blessings in your life and how achieving your goals will enhance your sense of gratitude and fulfillment.

3. Gratitude and Abundance Mindset:

An abundance mindset is the belief that there is more than enough to go around—that the universe is infinitely abundant and generous. Cultivating gratitude can shift us from a mindset of scarcity to one of abundance, helping us to see the limitless opportunities and possibilities that surround us.

Practice gratitude exercises such as abundance affirmations or visualization to cultivate an abundance mindset and attract more blessings into your life.

4. Gratitude and Emotional Intelligence:

Emotional intelligence is the ability to recognize, understand, and manage our own emotions as well as those of others. Cultivating gratitude can enhance our emotional intelligence by fostering greater empathy, compassion, and emotional resilience. When faced with challenging emotions, use gratitude as a tool to regulate your emotions and cultivate a sense of inner peace and well-being.

By integrating gratitude into our personal growth journey, we can unlock our full potential and create a life of deeper meaning, purpose, and fulfillment. As you continue on your path of self-discovery and transformation, may gratitude be your constant companion—a guiding light that illuminates the way forward and leads you to greater levels of joy, abundance, and fulfillment.

CHAPTER 5: SHARING AND AMPLIFYING GRATITUDE

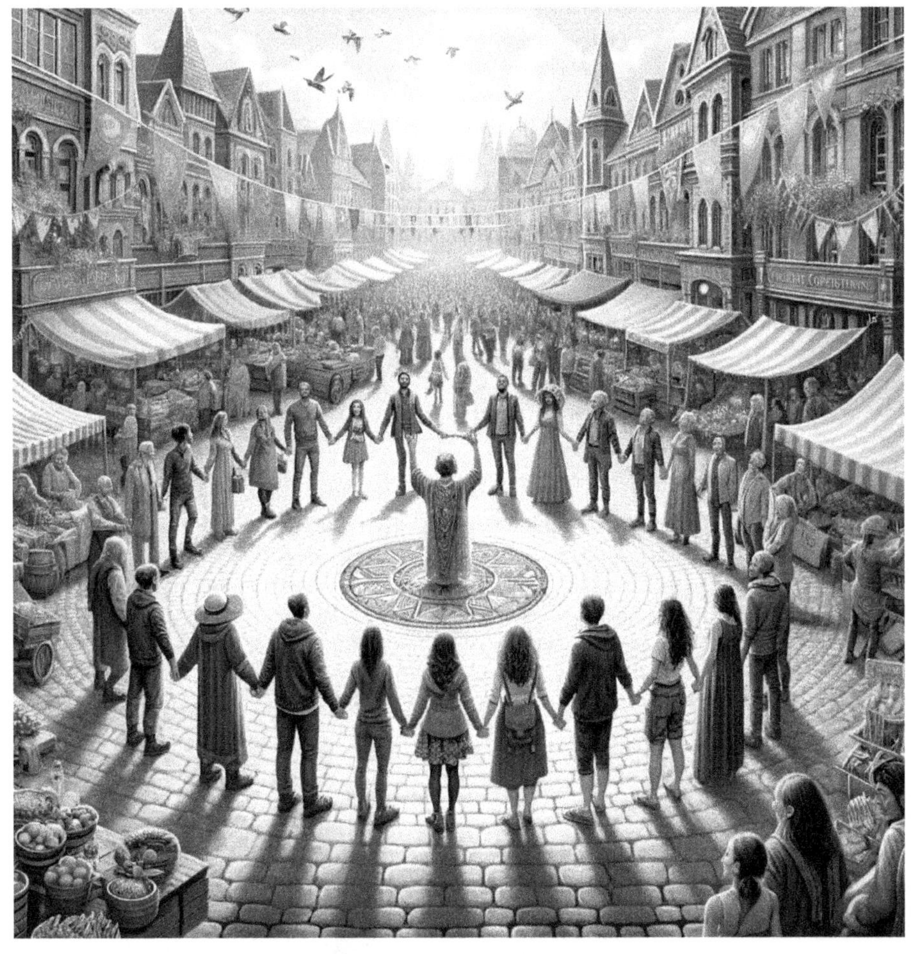

Gratitude has the remarkable ability to ripple outward, touching not only our own lives but also the lives of those around us. In this chapter, we will explore how sharing and amplifying gratitude can deepen our connections with others, foster a culture of appreciation, and magnify the positive impact of gratitude in our communities and workplaces.

1. Expressing Gratitude to Others:
One of the simplest yet most powerful ways to amplify gratitude is by expressing it to others. Take the time to sincerely thank the people in your life for their kindness, support, and contributions. Whether it's a heartfelt thank-you note, a verbal expression of appreciation, or a small act of kindness, expressing gratitude to others strengthens relationships, fosters connection, and spreads positivity.

2. Spreading Gratitude in Communities:
Gratitude has the power to create a ripple effect, spreading from person to person and radiating outward into our communities. Look for opportunities to spread gratitude in your community by participating in acts of kindness, volunteering your time and talents, or initiating gratitude-focused initiatives such as gratitude walks or community gratitude circles. By spreading gratitude in your community, you can help create a culture of appreciation and generosity that enriches the lives of everyone around you.

3. Gratitude in the Workplace:
The workplace is an ideal environment for cultivating gratitude and appreciation. Take proactive steps to foster a culture of gratitude in your workplace by recognizing and celebrating the

contributions of your colleagues, expressing appreciation for their hard work and dedication, and creating opportunities for gratitude to be expressed and acknowledged. A workplace culture that values gratitude fosters greater employee engagement, satisfaction, and well-being, leading to increased productivity and success for individuals and organizations alike.

4. Gratitude and Altruism:

Gratitude and altruism are deeply interconnected, each reinforcing and amplifying the other. Engage in acts of altruism and service to others as a way of expressing gratitude for the blessings in your own life. Whether it's volunteering your time, donating to a charitable cause, or simply offering a helping hand to someone in need, acts of altruism amplify the positive impact of gratitude and create a ripple effect of kindness and generosity that spreads far and wide.

By sharing and amplifying gratitude in our communities and workplaces, we can create a ripple effect of positivity and kindness that enriches the lives of everyone around us. As you seek out opportunities to express gratitude and spread kindness, may you be inspired by the transformative power of gratitude to create a world filled with compassion, connection, and abundance.

CHAPTER 6: SUSTAINING A GRATITUDE PRACTICE

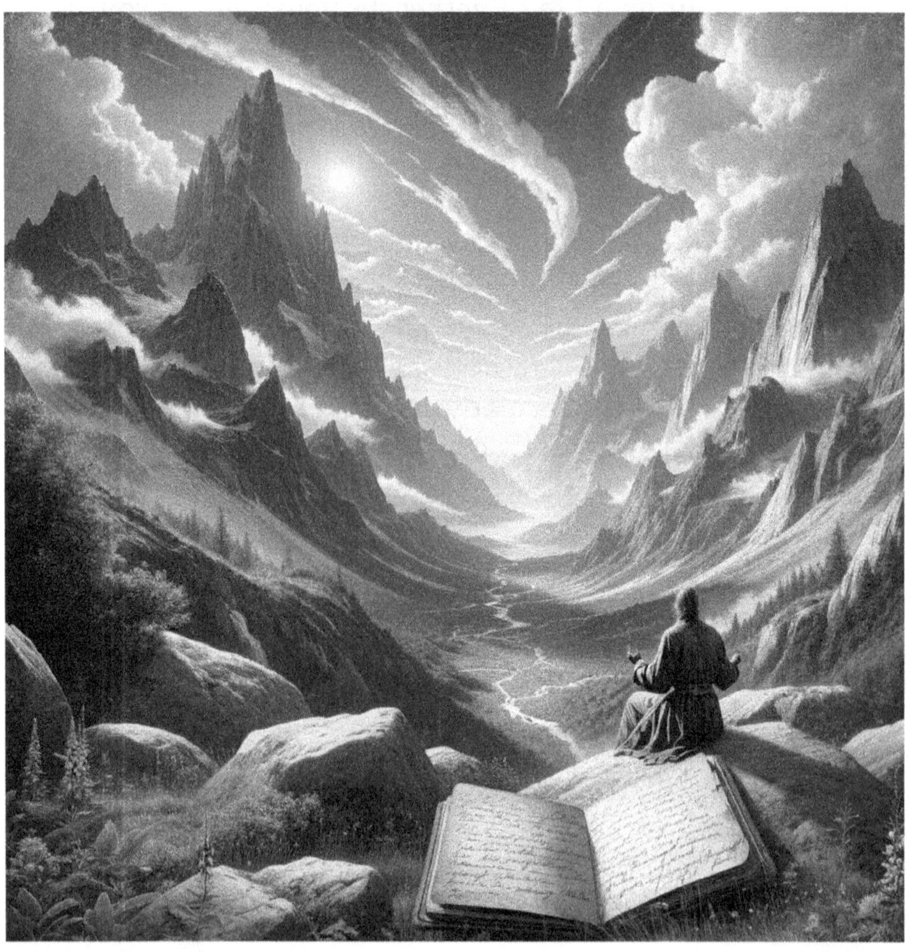

Cultivating gratitude is not a one-time endeavor but rather a lifelong journey—a continuous practice that requires dedication, intentionality, and commitment. In this chapter, we will explore strategies for sustaining a gratitude practice over the long term, overcoming challenges and setbacks, and deepening our appreciation for the abundance that surrounds us.

1. Overcoming Challenges and Setbacks:
Maintaining a gratitude practice may sometimes feel challenging, especially during times of difficulty or adversity. However, it is precisely during these times that practicing gratitude can be most beneficial. When faced with challenges or setbacks, remind yourself of the blessings in your life, no matter how small, and find moments of gratitude amidst the chaos. Use gratitude as a tool to anchor yourself in the present moment and cultivate resilience in the face of adversity.

2. Gratitude and Forgiveness:
Forgiveness is an essential aspect of sustaining a gratitude practice, both towards others and ourselves. Holding onto resentment or grudges can weigh us down and prevent us from fully embracing gratitude and appreciation. Practice forgiveness as a way of releasing negativity and opening your heart to the abundance of blessings that surround you. By letting go of past grievances and embracing forgiveness, you create space for gratitude to flourish and for new blessings to enter your life.

3. Gratitude as a Lifelong Journey:
Gratitude is not a destination to be reached but rather a journey to be embraced—a continuous process of growth, learning, and self-discovery. As you continue on your gratitude journey, be open to the ever-evolving nature of gratitude and the myriad ways in which it can enrich your life. Allow your gratitude practice

to evolve and adapt to the changing circumstances of your life, always remaining open to new experiences and opportunities for growth.

4. The Interconnectedness of Gratitude:

Gratitude is not just an individual practice but also a collective experience—a reminder of our interconnectedness and interdependence with all living beings. Recognize the ways in which your gratitude practice impacts not only your own life but also the lives of those around you. By cultivating gratitude, you contribute to a larger tapestry of kindness, compassion, and abundance that enriches the world and uplifts the human spirit.

As you embark on the journey of sustaining a gratitude practice, remember that you are not alone. Draw strength and inspiration from the collective wisdom and experiences of others who have walked this path before you. And above all, trust in the transformative power of gratitude to illuminate your life with joy, meaning, and fulfillment, now and for years to come.

Conclusion:

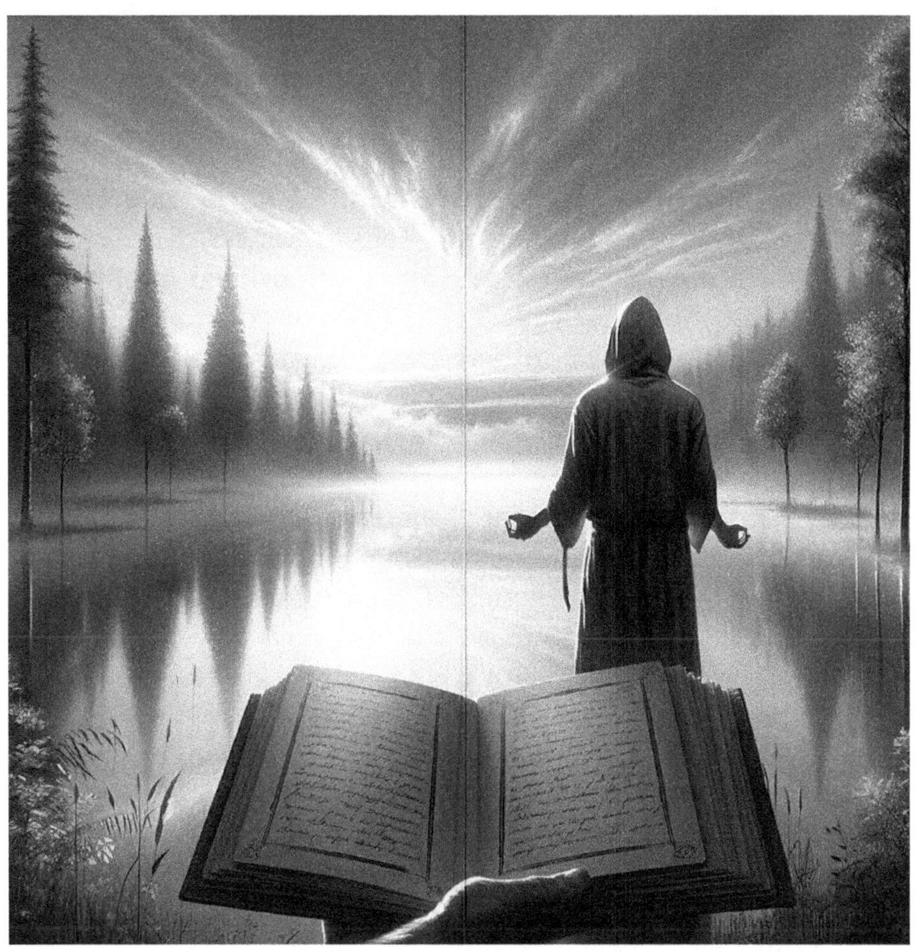

As we come to the end of "The Gratitude Journey: Discover, Embrace, and Flourish," let us pause to reflect on the profound lessons we have learned and the transformative power of gratitude that we have experienced.

Throughout this journey, we have explored the essence of gratitude—the deep-seated recognition of the abundance and beauty that surround us. We have delved into practical techniques and exercises for cultivating gratitude in our daily lives, from mindfulness practices to journaling, rituals, and expressions of appreciation. We have witnessed how gratitude can serve as a guiding light in the face of challenges, fostering resilience, and empowering us to find meaning and growth in even the darkest of times.

We have explored how gratitude can fuel our personal growth and development, enhancing our self-awareness, fostering an abundance mindset, and deepening our emotional intelligence. We have seen how gratitude has the power to ripple outward, touching the lives of others and creating a culture of kindness, compassion, and appreciation in our communities and workplaces.

And perhaps most importantly, we have come to understand that gratitude is not just a fleeting emotion but a lifelong journey—a continuous practice of mindfulness, reflection, and connection. As we continue on this journey, may we embrace the interconnectedness of all living beings and recognize the profound impact that our gratitude has on the world around us.
In closing, let us remember that gratitude is not a destination to be reached but a way of being—a fundamental orientation toward life that enriches every moment and infuses our existence with joy, meaning, and purpose. May you carry the lessons of gratitude with you always, allowing them to guide you on your journey toward a life of abundance, fulfillment, and flourishing.

Thank you for embarking on this journey with me. May your life be filled with gratitude, now and always.